Lower Your Cholesterol: 51 Proven Ways to Fight High Cholesterol

By Kiril Valtchev

Copyright 2016

Table of Contents

GENERAL INFORMATION

Before you can begin lowering your cholesterol, you need to first get a solid understanding of it. Let's get familiar with some of the general definitions:

1.) HDL

HDL stands for **High-Density Lipoproteins**. This is commonly known as **"good cholesterol"**. HDL's are one of the 5 major groups of lipoproteins. A HDL works by attaching itself to cholesterol and transporting it through your liver and out of your body. HDL's remove the fat molecules out of cells.

2.) LDL

LDL stands for **Low-Density Lipoproteins**. This is commonly known as **"bad cholesterol"**. This is the type of cholesterol that is harmful to have in your body. LDL's transfer fat around the body. They can clog the arteries and increase the risk of developing heart disease.

3.) THE RATIOS

Knowing the correct and healthy HDL and LDL ratios will help you be aware if you are at risk of being too high or too low. Below is breakdown of the levels:

Cholesterol Level	Category
Less than 200mg/dL	Good
200-239mg/dL	Borderline High
240mg/dL	High

LDL (Bad) Cholesterol Level	LDL Category
Less than 100 mg/dL	Optimal
100-129mg/dL	Near optimal/above optimal
130-159mg/dL	Borderline High
160-189mg/dL	High
190 mg/dL and up	Very High

HDL (Good) Level	HDL Category

Less than 40 mg/dL	A major risk factor for heart disease
40-59 mg/dL	The higher, the better
60 mg/dL and higher	Protective against heart disease

THE FOOD

Eating the right and healthy foods can greatly reduce your cholesterol levels. In this section we are going to list the different foods that can reduce your cholesterol.

4.) DIFFERENT OILS

There are many different types of cooking oils. Knowing which ones are healthy and which ones can be harmful is essential to having healthy cholesterol levels. Below is a list of the good oils and the bad oils:

Good Oils

- Coconut oil
- Olive oil
- Grapeseed oil
- Flax seed oil
- Extra-Virgin Olive oil

Bad Oils

- Corn oil
- Soybean oil
- Peanut oil
- Canola oil
- Cottonseed oil

5.) DARK CHOCOLATE

Yes. As much as this is a surprise dark chocolate can help reduce your cholesterol levels. On average people who eat a lot of cocoa powder and dark chocolate tend to have lower levels of bad LDL and 5% higher levels of good HDL.

6.) NUTS

Are you a person who loves nuts? Don't worry! Nuts (specifically almonds and walnuts) are not on the bad list of foods. A recent study has shown that eating 30 almonds a day for 1 month can reduce bad LDL cholesterol by 5% and raise good HDL cholesterol by 5%.

7.) EGGS

Eggs have always been a controversial topic in health awareness. Are eggs good for your or are they bad? Eggs are good for you, but they tend to be high in cholesterol. A large egg can contain up to 212 mg of cholesterol, which is very high compared to other foods. Eggs can raise your HDL. They can also change your LDL cholesterol from low to high. If you constantly eat eggs, it is good to pair them with low cholesterol foods for the rest of the day in order to have a healthy balance.

8.) POULTRY

For the most part, chicken and turkey tend to be low in saturated fat, especially when the skin is peeled off. This can greatly reduce the amount of cholesterol in meals. In general, red meat tends to have more cholesterol and saturated fat than chicken, fish, and vegetable proteins.

9.) READING MENUS

Today most restaurants have low fat and low cholesterol sections on their menus. If an option isn't listed on the menu, ask your waiter or waitress. Another option is to request smaller portions of your order or specifically ask the food to be prepared without foods that tend to be high in fat and cholesterol.

10.) INTELLIGENT SNACKING

It is very healthy to have small snacks throughout the course of a day. If you have small and proportional meals, it is good to eat small and healthy snacks throughout the day. Some of these include:

- Fruits
- Vegetables
- Pretzels
- Jam Yogurt
- Protein Trail Mix
- Pumpkin Seeds
- Popcorn

- Nutty Apples
- Smoothie
- Celery Sticks

11.) INTELLIGENT DESSERTS

It is good to treat yourself once in a while. There are actually some very health and low cholesterol deserts. Some of these include:

- Gelatin
- Frozen Yogurt
- Low Fat Pound Cake
- Banana Bread
- Peanut Butter Mousse (dairy-free)
- Rice Pudding
- Oat Squares
- Oatmeal Raisin Cookies
- Dried Cherry Pie
- Whole-Grain Cookies

12.) FIBER

Fiber is a great way to help your body keep you cholesterol levels down. Fiber helps your body wash away the bad cholesterol that gets stuck to the walls of your arteries. Soluble fiber not only helps to lower you cholesterol levels, but it also helps to regulate your blood sugar levels. Having a proportionate amount of fiber in your daily diet can reduce your cholesterol levels by close to 20% or more. Fiber can be found in some of the foods below:

- Avocados (11 grams per cup)
- Pears (10 grams of fiber)
- Brussel Sprouts (8 grams of fiber per cups)
- Black Beans (12 grams of fiber per cups)
- Chickpeas (8 grams of fiber per cup)

13.) GOOD BEANS

Healthy Beans can also help reduce your cholesterol levels. Beans are high in fiber and they are very effective in helping to lower your cholesterol because they contain **"pectin"**. Pectin is a fiber that helps to reduce blood cholesterol levels. Below are some examples of good beans:

- Lima Beans
- Kidney Beans
- Navy Beans
- Soybeans

14.) FISH

If you don't already have fish in your weekly diet it is important to start eating it. Eating fish two to three times per week instead of red meat can greatly reduce your cholesterol levels. Fish contains high levels of omega-3 fatty acids, which help to improve levels of HDL. Omega-3 fatty acids can also help to slow down the buildup of plaque in the arteries and reduce overall inflammation in the body.

15.) WHOLE GRAINS

Eating a higher amount of whole grains is an easy and healthy way to improve your cholesterol levels. A great way to control your cholesterol is by baking the food yourself. This way you know exactly what you are adding to the food. Below are a few examples of good whole grains to add to your diet:

- Whole Grain Bread
- Brown Rice
- Buckwheat
- Whole Rye
- Barley
- Quinoa
- 100% Whole Wheat Flour
- Wild Rice
- Oatmeal

16.) JUICES

Increasing the amount of juice you drink on a daily basis can also help lower your cholesterol. Juice can help to lower LDL. Fruits and vegetables contain high levels of antioxidants which aid in protecting the circulating cholesterol from oxidization. Oxidization is harmful to a person's health because it can elevate your blood pressure, harden your arteries and increases inflammation. Below are some healthy juice recipes that can help lower your cholesterol.

Peach Medley

- 2 Apples
- 10 Carrots
- 1 Lemon
- 1 Orange
- 2 peaches

Turmeric Sunrise

- 2 Apples
- 3 Carrots
- 3 Stalks of Celery
- 1 Thumb Ginger Root
- 2 Lemons
- 2 Pears
- 6 Thumb Turmeric Root

Heart Beet Root

- 1 Apple
- 1 Beet Root
- 12 Carrots
- ½ Lemon
- 2 Oranges

The Green Aid

- 4 Granny Smith Apples
- 3 Stalks of Celery
- 2 Leafs of Kale

- Lemon
- Spinach

Vegetable Blueberry

- 1 Apple
- 1 Cup Blueberries
- 1 stalk Broccoli
- 6 Carrots
- 1 Tomato

17.) MILK & CHEESE

 Milk and cheese in moderation can help reduce cholesterol. Cheese generally gets a bad rap because it tends to be high in saturated fat. Saturated fat is linked to increased levels of LDL. There are other arguments that cheese may not raise LDL. Milk is commonly perceived as a very healthy food, but it does contain high amounts of saturated fats. The higher the fat percentage in milk, the more it has the chance to raise your LDL. It really depends on how sensitive someone is to it. Below is small list of healthy milk and cheeses.

- Low-fat Cheese
- Low-fat Cottage Cheese
- Low-Fat Yogurt
- Skim or 1% Milk
- Almond Milk
- Non-fat yogurt

18.) OATMEAL

Eating oatmeal is not only a great way to start your breakfast, but it can bring down your LDL levels without bringing down your HDL levels. Oatmeal is high in soluble fiber which helps to lower your LDL levels. When oat fibers mix with cholesterol they end up carrying the cholesterol out of the body instead of allowing it to get absorbed into the blood stream.

19.) SWITCHING TO TEA

So why should you switch to tea? Standard teas and herbal teas are rich in antioxidants. The strength of the antioxidants depends on the type of tea, how it's processed and how it's prepared. The tea with the highest level of antioxidants is the hibiscus tea. You will not see drastic drops in your cholesterol from drinking tea only a few times. If you consistently drink tea throughout the week then you have a higher likelihood of noticing a decrease in your cholesterol levels. Below are some tea's that have been known to lower cholesterol.

- Green Tea
- Black Tea
- Peppermint Tea
- Red-bush Tea
- Ginger Tea

20.) HONEY

Does something as simple as honey lower cholesterol? The answer is yes. Honey is completely free of cholesterol. People have reported that having a small amount of honey in their daily diet can help keep cholesterol levels normal. Honey contains high levels of antioxidants, specifically darky honey. Honey is also high in minerals such as calcium, potassium, and sodium. Antioxidants in honey stop cholesterol from being moved out of the blood and into the inner lining of the blood vessels.

21.) FRUITS AND VEGETABLES

Do as your parents told you and eat your veggies! Fruits and vegetables are a great source to keep your cholesterol normalized. You should focus on eating 3-5 servings of fruits and vegetables a day. Below is a small list of fruits and vegetables you should add to your daily diet:

- Cabbage
- Avocado
- Blueberries
- Carrots
- Onions
- Grapes
- Soy beans
- Tomatoes
- Grapefruit

22.) BE CONSCIOUS OF TRANS-FAT FOODS

Trans-fat foods are foods that have unhealthy fat in them and can cause your cholesterol to increase. Below is small list of these foods.

- Cake Mix
- Donuts, cake, and pie
- Fast Food
- Dry Soup
- Energy Bars and Cereal Bars
- Biscuits
- Margarine
- Crackers
- Frozen Pizza

CONSISTENT EXERCISE

23.) YOGA

Practicing yoga 2-3 times per week is great way to regulate your cholesterol levels. Yoga has been known to improve blood and oxygen flow in the body. It helps to remove harmful toxins out of your body. Hot yoga is also a good way to regulate your cholesterol levels.

24.) LIFTING WEIGHTS

Can lifting weights help to lower your cholesterol? Lifting weights can help lower your LDL. Actually both your LDL and HDL can levels can improve when you lift weights. Consistent weight training can lower your body fat percentage and increase your lean body mass. Losing about 5% of your body fat can dramatically improve not only your cardiovascular health, but your cholesterol as well. The benefits of weight training are that your body will experience progressive improvement in your lipid profile and an overall reduction in your LDL.

25.) WALKING

Can something as simple as walking help you take control of your cholesterol? Walking is considered one of the lightest forms of exercise. Walking just 20-30 minutes per day can help improve your cardiovascular health and reduce your LDL by an average of 5-8%.

GO NATURAL

Vitamins, minerals and herbs can help you to regulate your cholesterol. It is important to incorporate a healthy balance of them into your diet. The key to maintaining a healthy cholesterol is a consistent and well balance diet. Having vitamins, minerals, and herbs in your diet can help you stay on a controlled balance with our cholesterol.

26.) VITAMIN C

Vitamin C is one of the best nutrients for the body. It is mostly associated with helping the body's immune system when a person has a cold. Below are some other benefits of vitamin C:

- Improves Immune System Deficiencies
- Fights Cardiovascular Disease
- Eye Disease
- Prenatal Health Issues
- Prevents skin wrinkling and slows down the aging process

27.) VITAMIN E

Supplements that contain different forms of vitamin E may reduce your cholesterol by almost 15% in people with high cholesterol. The most common form of vitamin E is **"tocopherol"**. Vitamin E is an antioxidant which helps to inhibit the oxidation of lipids and fatty acids. Below is a list of sources that contain vitamin E:

- Leafy Vegetables
- Pumpkin
- Spinach
- Whole Grain
- Avocado
- Corn

28.) PANTETHINE

Pantethine can reduce LDL-cholesterol while at the same time increasing HDL levels. You can take a supplement to get your dose of pantethine from some of the following foods below:

- Dairy
- Vegetables
- Salmon
- Grains
- Meat
- Yeast
- Liver
- Eggs

29.) Calcium

Clinical trials have shown that calcium can help reduce cholesterol. There are many health benefits of having calcium in your diet, such as the strengthening of bones. So how does calcium lower your cholesterol? It is not 100% clear. The way calcium works is by binding to bile acids and cholesterol in the small intestine. By binding to cholesterol in the small intestine, cholesterol is not absorbed directly into the blood stream and is instead excreted out of the body in the poop. Below are some foods that provide a great source of calcium:

- Milk
- Cheese
- Broccoli
- Sardines
- Kale

30.)CHROMIUM

What is chromium? Chromium is a mineral that is used by our bodies to aid in normal body functions, like food digestion. It helps to control your blood sugar, cholesterol and fat metabolism. Low levels of chromium can increase your blood sugar levels, cholesterol levels and other conditions, such as diabetes and heart disease. Below is a list of foods that have good sources of chromium:

- Cheese
- Yeast
- Lean Meat
- Whole Grain

31.) ARTICHOKE EXTRACT

Artichoke extract can help reduce your cholesterol levels. In clinical trials it's been proven to lower cholesterol by nearly 15%. You can read more about it here: http://www.webmd.com/vitamins-supplements/ingredientmono-842-artichoke.aspx?activeingredientid=842

32.) POLICOSANOL

What is policosanol? Policosanol is a mixture of alcohols extracted from plant waxes. It is mainly used as a dietary supplement. It reduces cholesterol production in the liver and helps to break down LDL cholesterol. It also helps to reduce blood clots. Below are some foods that contain policosanol:

- Yams
- Sugar Cane
- Wheat
- Beeswax

33.) BETA GLUCAN

What is Beta Glucan? Beta glucan is a type of sugar that is found in the cell walls of bacteria, yeast, fungi and other plants such as barley and oats. They are used to help regulate high cholesterol, diabetes, cancer and even HIV/AIDS. The beta-glucan works by forming a layer in the small intestine.

It aids in the re-absorption of bile acids, which the body makes from cholesterol. It absorbs the current cholesterol that circulates around the body and uses it to make new bile acids. Since it uses the cholesterol to produce new bile acids this results in reduced cholesterol levels. Below are some foods that contain beta glucan:

- Barley
- Oats
- Seaweed
- Mushrooms

34.) B VITAMINS

B Vitamins are also another great way to lower your cholesterol. B vitamins have been commonly known as energy vitamins. They help your body obtain energy from the food you consume. They help to lower your LDL cholesterol levels while increasing your HDL levels. Below is the family of B-vitamins:

- B1, B2, B3, B5, B6, B12

35.) SOY ISOFLAVONES

What are soy isoflavones? Soy isoflavones are phytochemicals that are found only in plants. They are a type of plant hormone that is similar to human estrogen. They can help lower your LDL levels and raise your HDL levels at the same time. They help prevent the buildup of plaque in your arteries and stop blood clots from forming. They are most concentrated in soybeans.

36.) BETA SITOSTEROL

Beta sitosterol is taken to help moderate your cholesterol levels. It is most commonly found in plants such as fruits, vegetables, seeds and nuts. It helps to fight against colon cancer, allergies, cervical cancer, hair loss, chronic fatigue, common cold and much more.

37.) RED YEAST EXTRACT

Red yeast extract is another way to lower your cholesterol. It is typically sold as digestive supplement. It is a powder that is extracted from fermented dried rice. It is most commonly used in China as a way to lower your cholesterol.

38.) GUGGULIPIDS

What the heck are guggulipids? Despite having an odd name, guggulipids are one of the best supplements to lower your cholesterol. It's a herb from India that has been used as a natural remedy for centuries. It is extracted from a special type of tree known as a myrrh tree that is found in India. Below are other things that guggulipids help to heal:

- Arthritis
- Obesity
- Stomach ulcers

39.) JIAOGULAN

This natural herb helps to reduce the production of LDL cholesterol. It is a plant that grows in China and has been used for many years as an antioxidant herb and illness- prevention remedy. It contains healthy minerals such as amino acids, proteins and B vitamins. It reduces cholesterol by improving how the liver sends sugar and carbs to the muscles to convert energy instead of storing the sugar as fat.

40.) OTHER COMMONLY KNOWN HERBS

There are a lot of different herbs and remedies that can also lower your cholesterol. Below are some more:

- Ginger
- Turmeric
- Green Tea
- Licorice Extract
- Holy Basil
- Yarrow
- Rosemary

MEDICATION

Not everyone will be able to lower their cholesterol with diet and exercise. Sometimes it is best to visit your doctor and get more information on other alternatives. There is certain medication that can be taken to help reduce your cholesterol levels.

41.) STATINS

Statins block the production of cholesterol in the liver and intestines. Below are some commonly known drugs that do the trick.

- Lipitor
- Crestor
- Lescol
- Mevacor
- Zocor
- Pravachol

42.) NICOTINIC ACID

Nicotinic acid is just a high dose of B vitamins. They are typically prescribed by a doctor. Below are some examples:

- Niaspan
- Nicolar

43.) FIBRATES

What are fibrates? They help to reduce the amount of non-fatal heart attacks. They are less effective when it comes to lowering your LDL, but are very affective in increasing your HDL. Below are commonly prescribed fibrates.

- Modalim
- Lopid
- TriCor
- Lipoclin
- Bezalip

44.) BILE ACID SEQUESTRANTS

According to WebMD, sequestrants bind to bile acids in the intestine and prevent them from being absorbed in the blood stream. The liver then produces more bile to replace the bile that has been lost during this process. Since the body requires cholesterol to make bile, the liver uses the cholesterol in the blood which ends up reducing the amount of LDL cholesterol that circulates in the blood. Below are some common bile acid sequestrants.

- Colestid
- Welchol
- Locholest
- Prevalite

45.) EZETIMIBE

Ezetimibe works by reducing the amount of cholesterol that your body absorbs. It has been known to reduce your LDL cholesterol up to 20%.It lowers your plasma cholesterol levels. Below are some commonly known drugs:

- Zetia
- Ezetrol
- Vytorin
- Inegy

CONCLUSION

Lowering your cholesterol is a matter of developing consistent daily habits. It should be a healthy balance of diet and exercise. You should focus on a long term approach to balancing a healthy cholesterol level.

46.) LOSE WEIGHT

Losing weight is the most straightforward way to naturally reduce your cholesterol levels. Low to moderate exercise 2-3 times per week can help raise your HDL and lower your LDL cholesterol. By having a consistent exercise schedule you can sustain a healthy and balanced weight. This will help to moderate your cholesterol and keep it at healthy levels.

47.) SELF EDUCATION

The amount of information about your overall health and cholesterol can be found all over the internet. Below are some good sources.

- WebMD
- Wikipedia
- Local Library
- Health Newsletters

48.)STOP SMOKING

Smoking is very harmful to a person's health. Quitting smoking can help lower your cholesterol. Smoking has been known to raise your LDL cholesterol and lower your HDL cholesterol. It may be hard for people to quit smoking, but if you have high cholesterol smoking will only make it worse.

49.)STRESS MANAGEMENT

Stress can have a very negative effect on your overall health. Anxiety and pressure can shift your hormones out of a healthy balance and cause your cholesterol to spike up. It can drastically increase your LDL levels. If you are highly anxious and stressed out person you should begin to concentrate on ways to reduce your stress levels. Below are a few methods:

- Drink a glass of wine

- Eat Dark Chocolate
- Meditation
- Socialize with Friends

50.)THYROID CHECK

If your cholesterol still continues to stay at a high level, you should go to your doctor and get your thyroid examined. A low thyroid level can cause your LDL cholesterol to increase and cause you to be severely tired. If you are over the age of 40, it is good to get your thyroid examined at least once a year.

51.)BECOME COMMITTED

Your cholesterol isn't going to magically get better. It is up to you to make a solid commitment to bring it back to healthy levels. Create a consistent daily diet and exercise regimen and follow it consistently. Your cholesterol is something that is completely manageable if you truly care about your well-being. Take the necessary steps outlined in this guide and you will have positive results.